Touched

True Stories From Inside The Massage Room

Kamillya Hunter

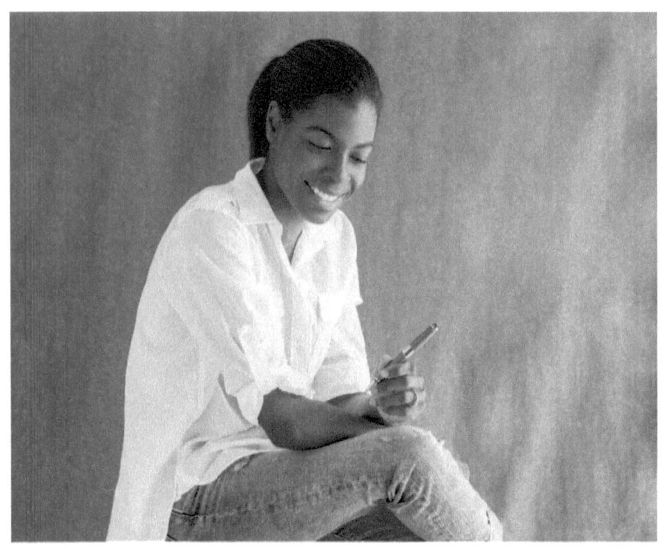

KAMILLYA HUNTER is a self-diagnosed spa junkie. She is originally from Joliet, Illinois and a proud graduate of The Ohio State University. Hunter is also the author of Success Of A Failed Therapist: A motivational and professional resource to the massage therapist.

TOUCHED

DEDICATION

This is dedicated to the clients who trusted me with their bodies, the massage therapists who give of themselves unselfishly, the Unicorns who discovered the importance of frequent bodywork, and to my fellow black bodyworkers, you are not alone.

CONTENTS

ACKNOWLEDGMENTS

The biggest thank you goes to my husband, Hakeem, and my best friend, Shira, for your unending support. Thank you for listening, reading, and believing in everything I do. And to my editor, Paula Lester, for helping me pick up the words and put them in all the right places.

MY ADDICTION

KAMILLYA HUNTER

It's amazing when you think about how many people feel guilty for getting such a necessary service as massage. Touch is necessary. Remove all thoughts of luxury for a moment and think about the basic need for touch. From birth, infants are soothed by touch. Adults use touch as a form of nonverbal communication to express affection, comfort, anger, and many other emotions. It's been researched at length by experts in the fields of psychology, neuroscience, and more.

I never received massage prior to diving head first into school for it. It just seemed like a cool thing to do after I'd dropped out of college with no future plans. When I finally received one, a professional massage, I was introduced to an addiction I never knew existed.

My career as a licensed massage therapist began at the young age of twenty-two. For years, I bounced around, searching for the right environment for me. My journey began in a chiropractic office, which left me jaded and emotionally scarred. From there, I worked in just about every type of environment imaginable: small massage clinics, fitness centers, country clubs, luxury spas, franchises, hotels, and eventually my own private practice. It wasn't until I transitioned out of the treatment room that I was able to reflect back upon my experiences as a massage therapist and try and make sense of them all.

It was years before I began to appreciate all the physical and emotional benefits massage could bring to both my clients and me. I was helping people heal from chronic pain, providing relief to mothers growing new babies, and allowing others to escape the stress of everyday life, even if only for one hour.

I eventually learned that massage was much more than a job that put food on my table. Throughout my career, I met and touched thousands of people. Many only came across my table once, and I saw others too many times to count. The following clients left a permanent impression on my life, whether they realized it or not. These are the stories that helped me realize that the power of touch is never delivered in just one direction. They are in no particular order. The names have been changed to protect their privacy.

THE UNICORN

I put in a two-week notice with my job at the call center immediately after I secured the massage position at the family-owned chiropractic office. I was eager to finally escape the collection agency that robbed me of the compassion I had for others. I put my notice in the moment my new employer asked, "When can you start?"

At the chiropractic office, my patients only received a 15-minute session before it was the doctor's turn to give them an adjustment. The patient's time with the doctor was usually less than five minutes, and it was my job to relax them before he took them back. That meant poking and prodding them through layers of clothing, searching for knots and chronic pain points that had been bothering them for years. The experience was damaging to my thumbs, wrists, and most of all, my ego.

I doubted I would be able to offer any relief during such short amounts of time. It was possible I could do more to help my patients, but I needed more time and a proper setting to exercise the skills I had learned in school. The patients who did receive full 30- and 60-minute sessions were loyal to the other two massage therapists on staff, and none of them wanted to book with me, especially when they found out I was new.

A position in a medical office wasn't my dream job. I wanted luxury, soft music, and dimly lit rooms. I wanted my patients and myself to be greeted with the smell of lavender and other heavenly essential oil blends. The medical office offered the choice between Lysol and diluted bleach water. I wanted clients, not patients. I wanted tips, not medical charts. The chiropractic office was everything I never wanted and then some. There wasn't even privacy. Except for the full sessions, the massages all happened right out in the open. My patients never needed to get undressed, so no one seemed to be bothered by the lack of privacy except me.

One day, after I had been on the job for nearly two weeks, the receptionist retrieved me from the break room, informing me that a unicorn had scheduled a full hour session and volunteered to "try me out." I didn't try to hide my excitement. This was my chance to show off those techniques I had spent the past year mastering, a chance to give a *real* massage. I quickly raced to find an empty treatment room. There were only two rooms, and one was in use by a seasoned therapist who had been working there for six years. She was always booked solid. The other room was right next to it, and the door was wide open. I peeked inside to give it a quick inspection and to make sure the table was set, the light was on, and everything was in place.

I headed to the lobby and was formally introduced to a large man who was three times my size, twice my age, and quite overdressed for the occasion. He wore a full suit and shoes that probably cost more than my entire month's pay. The only thing we had in common was the color of our skin.

He smiled, shook my hand, and gave me a look that let me know he was pleased to meet a massage therapist of color. It was a look that I had come to recognize, even in my brief experience working in the field. Apparently, black massage therapists were like mythical creatures that only existed in fairy tales, only I didn't know it at the time. I did know that black clients were rare. It turned out we were just as few and far between as they were. I later discovered that the chance meeting between a black client and a black therapist happened so infrequently that I welcomed each encounter with a desire to leave everything on the table, hoping they would realize the benefits of bodywork and return as often as the majority.

The unicorn followed quietly behind me as I led him to the treatment room. When we arrived, I began the interview.

"Have you had a massage before?"

"Girl, I've had more massages than you've given. Just do your thang, and I'll let you know if I don't like it." I was so overly confident that I ignored the condescension in his tone. I didn't want to offend him or embarrass myself any further.

"Okay. Sounds good to me." It was a terrible first client interview, considering I only asked one question. Over time, my client interviews, or intakes as we refer to them in the industry, became so automated that I could go through the entire script without stopping to take a breath.

I stepped out of the room so he could undress in private. It was my first full session, so I was a bit rusty at estimating the amount of time a client needed to get undressed.

While in school, there was a woman who arrived ten minutes late to her massage appointment. When she finally did get there, she spent another two minutes shouting at the receptionist after being informed that she would not receive her full time on the table.

"I'll try to give you as much time as possible. If we head back now, we can get a good 45 minutes in." It was my best attempt at de-escalating the situation. With massage, every minute counts so I wanted to hurry her along.

"Are *you* doing my massage?"

"Yes, I'll be your therapist today. Would you like to head back?"

"Are you strong? You don't look strong. I like deep tissue. You look too skinny to be strong enough for what I need," she barked as we headed down the hall to the room.

"I'm pretty strong. Just let me know about the pressure when we begin the massage, and I can try to adjust for you."

Growing up, I was always teased by my family for being thin. I never imagined I would be openly shamed to my face for being too thin to deliver a good enough massage. But that was only the beginning of the onslaught.

When we made it to the room, my client began immediately undressing right in front of me. She was possibly in her mid-60s. Time and gravity had not been kind. It was not a body I wanted to see without clothes. I insisted that she wait for me to finish her interview so I could step out of the room to give her privacy.

"Just get out and don't go far! I only need a second, so don't go anywhere!" Whatever caused this woman to be late for the appointment must have stayed with her and ruined her whole day. At least, that is what I needed to tell myself to help me power through her session.

I left the room as quickly as I could and headed to the bathroom to wash my hands. In past appointments, my clients had complained of my hands being cold. Because of that, I made certain to warm my massage lotion in the microwave. A 20-second burst usually did the trick. Any longer and the lotion would either be too wet or too hot to use

While I was heading back down the hall toward

the room, I heard shouting. I could not believe my ears.

"I'M READY! I'M READY! I'M READYYYYYYY!"

The receptionist rushed down the hall. Two other massage students opened their doors and poked their heads out to see what was going on. I tapped on the door and stepped quickly inside, hoping it would diffuse her anger.

"Girl, are you deaf? You didn't hear me shouting I was ready?"

"I needed to wash my hands."

"I better not get shorted any time! I was ready and you were off somewhere when I told you not to go far."

This client spent the better half of the remaining time in her session telling me how I wasn't doing it right. She mentioned that there was another therapist there who was better than anyone else she'd tried. We were all students, so the clinic was meant for us to gain hands-on experience with real, paying clients. The therapist she preferred was nearing graduation and that meant she was more experienced than me.

After the massage, I met the client outside the room with a cup of water.

"I don't want that!" she said as she waved her hand and stormed up the hall. "I didn't get my whole time. I'm not paying for that!" I could hear her shouting at the receptionist, who insisted the loss of time was due to her late arrival.

In truth, I had cut her session short. My patience for her treatment of me in the room had been worn out. It was one of the worst massages I had ever given. The following week, the woman returned in the sweetest mood. She was booked again with the therapist she loved and all was right again in her world.

After some time had passed, I knocked gently and entered the room, ready to begin the unicorn's massage. I quickly realized that I had made a rookie mistake. I had forgotten to lower my table. I prayed he wouldn't ask for more pressure because he was a pretty big guy and I couldn't go that deep without using my full bodyweight. The request would be out of the question because the table was too high.

The small talk began the moment I entered the room. I found out he was a former professional athlete who was a local celebrity. If he hadn't mentioned it, I would not have known. Aside from barely watching his sport, I wasn't from the city or state of his self-proclaimed fame. His name and status meant nothing to me. Judging from his size and build, I could have guessed it was the case, but I was still new to this and hadn't seen many different body types.

I worked my way through his neck to one arm and then headed around to the other side of the table to begin working on the other. *Ah, second rookie mistake.* I'd left my massage lotion on the other side of the room. My flow was interrupted. His hand brushed against my hip when I walked around the table. *My mistake,* I thought. He was a relatively big guy. After all, he was a former pro athlete and our standard massage tables didn't exactly support a wider frame. It was very common for people's arms to hang over the sides, even while they were face-up on the table.

I retrieved my lotion bottle and made an extra effort to step widely around his hand. As I massaged his arm, I noticed him rubbing my leg with the back of his hand. I hoped it was only involuntary muscle contractions because I was massaging his arm. Using one hand, I lifted, rotated, and pinned his arm on the table and then continued massaging his bicep with the other.

Suddenly, he mentioned he was a bit warm. Before I could respond, he removed the top blanket and tossed it carelessly onto the floor. He lowered the thin top sheet, folded it down very low at his waist, and breathed a deep sigh of relief.

"Can I get you some water?"

"No, this is fine."

I continued to his legs.

"Do you only work here?"

"For massage? Yes, but I also work for a call center." I only had a few more days at the call center, but he didn't need to know that.

"Do you visit homes?"

"No. My table doesn't fit in my tiny car."

"I'm sure you could make it work. I prefer to get

massages at home."

"I'm comfortable just working here."

"You could make way more money. We could just make a pallet on the floor and that would work fine."

"Nah. I'm comfortable just working here." I tried to act oblivious at his attempt to solicit more than a massage. I didn't like confrontation or making others uncomfortable, so it was better to act clueless than to make the situation worse.

It didn't take long to determine that the touches he was delivering to me were intentional and my gut was right. I rushed through the massage of his second leg while he made numerous comments about his teenage daughter being gone for most of the day and how the sessions would be private if I came to his home. I hurried to turn him over and prayed this would put an end to the conversation. With his face down in the cradle, I began to hate the fact that there was a hole for him to breathe.

The one-sided conversation continued, and it became clear that the problem was not that his arms and hands were just too big to fit comfortably at his sides. He conveniently lifted them as I walked by and attempted to touch my legs. The size of the room made it a bit difficult to step beyond his reach, but my small frame helped. Things got trickier when I needed to stand at the side of the table for a longer period of time to massage his back. After he landed a few successful gropes, I discovered a useful trick. I lifted his arm onto the table and tucked the sheet tightly under and around his hand. His arm was locked securely in place with the sheet. In that moment, I was proud of myself for finding a non-confrontational solution to the problem.

Finally, the session was over.

"Alright Mr. Unicorn. We're all done. Take as much time as you need getting up, and I'll get you some water."

"Thanks, girl. That was great." He raised his body up with his arms, rolled over, and stood at the side of the table, fully exposed. "Leave me your number, and I'll make sure to book the next ones directly with you."

For the life of me, I can't explain how I stood there long enough for him to speak. Maybe it was shock, possibly fear. It was definitely inexperience. I managed to calmly and politely decline the invitation to be his personal masseuse. I pretended to be unaware of his advances.

"Oh, I'm sorry. Let me step out so you can have some privacy to get dressed." I waited for what felt like an eternity outside the door. I thanked him for coming and gestured him to the front so he could check out.

I re-entered the room and collected the sheets on the table, along with the blanket that was thrown on the floor. I walked across the hall to shove them into the stacked washer. When I withdrew my arm, I felt cold, wet fluid drag across my arm. I knew immediately what it was.

Disgusted, I ran to my treatment room, closed the door, and headed straight to the sink in the corner. I began layering handfuls of liquid soap onto my hands and arms, all the way up to my elbows. Layer, scrub, rinse, repeat. Layer, scrub, rinse, repeat. In case you were wondering, no amount of scrubbing could remove the layers of violation I felt.

I still had not turned the room. The next therapist began gently but persistently tapping on the door. She finally opened it and mumbled, "Seriously?" beneath her breath. It was five minutes past when her session was supposed to begin. I tried to apologize for making her late. She didn't look at me, nor did she attempt to hide her annoyance. "This isn't just your room, you know. If you're going to be doing full sessions, you need to end *on time*," she grumbled as she quickly put fresh sheets on the table. "It's unprofessional and disrespectful to make me late for my client just because you don't know how to end on time."

Trying to explain the reason I was running behind would have done me no good. She was in no mood to hear it, and I didn't know where to begin. I had never imagined I would be scrubbing seminal fluid from my arm after my first full session at a real job. They don't tell you this in school.

I thanked the other therapist for making the table. She rolled her eyes and forced out a sarcastic "Thanks." She turned the corner and greeted her client in the sweetest way possible. It was sort of like a Jekyll to the Hyde-like encounter I had just had with her. It was a skill I learned to master over time. Clients should never be aware of drama happening behind the scenes. Fake smiles, friendly hellos, and reflexive apologies were things I learned would keep my tips high and my books full.

I headed to the break room and there stood the unicorn, chatting it up with the chiropractor. The unicorn smiled at me in a way that made me feel small, like a child. Maybe that's how he saw me, as a naïve child. He was wrong. After a few minutes of familiar banter with his lifelong friend, the unicorn finally left.

I pulled the chiropractor aside and told him I had felt very uncomfortable in that session. I was certain the unicorn was overly flirtatious and that he'd intentionally touched me at times. My concerns were met with denial.

"I've known him for years. He's happily married, with a family." The chiropractor, my employer, completely dismissed my complaint. He chalked it up to me being green and lacking experience with working on male clients.

"Is it okay if he's not booked with me again?" I requested sheepishly, tears starting to fill my eyes.

"That's fine, but he really enjoyed your massage. We're trying hard to build your books. No one wants to try you because you're new. He did!" He stormed off toward the front and told the receptionist, "Don't book her with any more full sessions."

"But Mr. Unicorn scheduled again for next week," the receptionist replied.

"Move him to someone else. She said she's not ready for full sessions."

The other massage therapist was upset with me for causing her to be late. While I waited in the break room for another 15-minute patient, I overheard her venting to the other seasoned therapist. "If she can't stay on time, she doesn't need to be given full sessions. When I went into the room, she wasn't even making the table. She was just standing there, taking her time, washing her hands in the sink."

"See, that's why he shouldn't have hired somebody right out of school. I think he was just desperate. We're busy but not *that* busy. You and I can handle it," the other therapist replied.

I left work that day feeling ashamed and guilty for not being appreciative of the only client who was willing to give me a chance. I questioned whether I'd overreacted and misunderstood what had happened. I wondered if my memory was replaying only the negative and exaggerating the experience. The next day, I was fired for not being a good fit.

It was the first time I had been fired from a job. Other than the chiropractor, I never told anyone what happened, but this became the moment that shaped the rest of my experiences inside the massage room.

DR. JEKYLL AND MRS. HYDE

Most of my regulars made small talk with me. They would chat about how someone at work had upset them or how traffic had been a bear that day. Maybe *everything* was going wrong for them, and they were looking forward to their time with me.

But not Dr. Jekyll.

He was one of the quiet ones. These were people who would often want to see me frequently, even flipping out if they couldn't get onto my table. But once they got there, they didn't chat with me like most of my clients did.

Dr. Jekyll never said a word outside of telling me the body areas he wanted me to work. His sessions were always silent aside from the massage music playing softly from the CD player.

Quiet ones like him were actually the clients I loved most, the ones who let me take control of their sessions. They let me determine the pressure, and they didn't interrupt with weird sounds or annoying requests.

I liked to approach every massage like I would a blank canvas, letting my hands go where-ever they needed to, making long, beautiful stokes. When I massaged, I saw colors. Shades of blues, pinks, and purples swirled before me. I could see the energy flowing from my hands through their bodies, and it continued on from there. I removed the negative energy and tossed it out into the universe, away from their bodies and mine. I had figured out how to ground myself before a massage. I knew how to put a wall up at the level of my wrists, so I wouldn't absorb the issues I was removing from the client on my table.

Dr. Jekyll was the client I needed. Every two weeks, he was a new, blank canvas who never said a word. He just came in and let me do what I did best: amazing Swedish massage.

Most therapists look down their noses at colleagues who love to give relaxing massages. "Fluff and buff," is what the industry would call it, but I never cared. It was my specialty.

Months passed, and since Dr. Jekyll never told me about his life, I created one for him in my mind. I threw my hands on autopilot with the music and envisioned him at his job. His shoulder muscles told me he worked at a computer all day. He was thin and of average height. I imagined that he woke up every morning at 5 am to go for an early morning jog. He'd return home to shower before his wife and children awoke.

By 7 am, his wife would have already made

breakfast, dressed the children, and ushered them off to the bus stop. He would leave the house around 8 am for a 45-minute commute to work. If he left much after that, he'd risk being late, and his boss would have none of that. He worked in statistical data entry because what could be more boring than that? He ate the same uninspiring ham and cheese sandwich every day, alone at his desk.

He wasn't very social at work. Although he held a PhD in statistics, he never got the positions he wanted because he just wasn't aggressive enough. So there he sat, day after day, in the same cubicle, eating the same sandwich, and following the same daily routine. He needed his massage to be a specific way each time because his entire life was a routine.

His skin was smooth, and he didn't have much body hair. It wasn't something I had noticed during the first few months I saw him, but his legs were very smooth. In fact, they were smoother than those of any male client I had ever had. I created a new story in my mind. He was now a swimmer but not a professional one. Better yet, Dr. Jekyll was a math teacher who coached the swim team after school. He kept his legs smooth because it helped him be faster in the water. He needed massage to work out the cramps in his legs from doing too many laps in the pool.

While Dr. Jekyll didn't have much body hair, I began to notice that he was letting the hair on his head grow long. It was actually longer than the hair of any male professor or teacher I'd ever known, so I had to change his life in my mind again. He was now in a garage band with some old high school buddies, and they had gigs on the weekends. He was reliving his youth during a mid-life crisis. He needed massage to help get the creative juices flowing for the new songs he wanted to create. He never spoke to me because he was saving his voice for the weekends.

One day, Dr. Jekyll asked me to schedule his next session under the name "Mrs. Hyde," and I obliged, never asking why.

During Mrs. Hyde's first session, she cried. I offered her a cup of water, and she graciously accepted. I gave her some tissue. She wiped her eyes, dabbed her nose, laid back, and allowed me to continue the massage. She never said a word. She sniffled a few times but that was all.

Over the next few months, I began creating a life for Mrs. Hyde. She was a spy. When she was caught, she escaped from the prison where the enemies locked her away. She used her stealth and skills to sneak past the unsuspecting guards and free herself.

Her arms and legs were much more muscular than those of any other woman I had worked on in the past. She was now a gymnast. Back in her earlier days, she had competed in the junior Olympics, narrowly missing the medal every time. It was the balance beam that always got her. She kept at it anyway, training harder and harder each year. Finally, she took third, which was her own personal best. The medal still hangs in a case above her fireplace.

The stubble on Mrs. Hyde's face pricked my fingers as I closed out our final massage. The tears had dried, her sinuses were clear, and she finally spoke to me, thought it was only two words. "Thank you."

All of the lives I had imagined had been wrong or at least only partial. My client had come to see me during her gender transition. Dr. Jekyll had become Mrs. Hyde, and she stopped coming in to see me after that. I guess she didn't need massage anymore. I hope I helped her through a difficult time and gave her space to think and just be, without having every moment filled with words.

SAY SOMETHING

Sometimes underage clients would have a parent in the room. Sometimes a mother would bring her child into the room. For me, as long as the other person was not disruptive, taking photos or videos, and was physically out of my way, I didn't care.

Some therapists disagree, and for good reason. There are some people who are aroused by massage and watching a massage fulfills a fantasy of some sort for them. After ten years in the industry, there are very few things I haven't encountered, but that is one.

But there was a client who began coming to me at the strong recommendation of her boyfriend. He came with her to the first appointment, and she was noticeably uncomfortable. He requested to be in the room during the treatment. This was the first time I'd had a significant other request to sit in on a massage. Using this as an opportunity to exercise great customer service skills, I granted him access to the treatment room, as long as it was okay with her. She seemed reluctant but agreed.

I led them both back to the treatment room and motioned him to the single client chair in the far corner of the room. Some massage rooms are extremely small. Fortunately, this wasn't one of them. It wasn't the largest room I had worked in—it couldn't fit two tables for a couple's massage, but there was more than enough room for the three of us. Besides, she would be on the table.

The size of this room would make any massage therapist feel spoiled in that there was ample room to walk comfortably around the table without fear of tripping, rubbing the wall, or high-stepping over the corner of the massage table. I've worked in a room that small, and it is not ideal. Had this room been of that size, the answer to his request would have definitely been no. Thinking back, I guess I could have told him the treatment room wouldn't be big enough for him to chaperone her massage, but I saw no harm in his request.

I did my usual intake while completely ignoring him in the corner. He seemed okay enough. He just sat quietly. Didn't ask any questions. Didn't make any weird requests. He just sat there. During the session, he never spoke. Neither did she. When I asked about pressure, she said it was fine and that was all. I try not to engage in conversation unless the client initiates. And even then, I try to keep talk focused on the massage.

The session came and went. Honestly, I forgot he was even there. They rescheduled the following week and that was that.

The next week came, and they both arrived. I assumed he wanted to sit in again, and I was correct. She still appeared reluctant and annoyed that he wanted to be in the room, but it wasn't my battle to fight. If she didn't want her boyfriend in the room, she could simply say so, and I would decline the request. She mumbled a comment about him just being jealous as she headed back to my room. He took his normal place in the corner. This time, he came prepared with headphones. I guess the lulling sound of spa music wasn't to his liking.

While working on her arms, I noticed a few bruises on her wrists and one of her biceps. I specifically asked if the pressure was okay when I got to those areas, and she said it was fine. But what I saw when I undraped her legs was nothing I had ever seen before. There were dark purple bruises all over her legs. For the first time, I was very aware of his presence in the room.

Growing up, I had witnessed domestic abuse. A high school friend of mine was raped, set on fire, and thrown in a dumpster by her boyfriend, who was 10 years older than her.

My dad's cousin, who we called "aunt," was murdered by her boyfriend, who later fled and spent years on the run. I remember that, when the police finally caught him, my dad and grandmother made the front page of our local newspaper.

With those thoughts in mind, I began to fear my

client's life. Ideas of how those bruises had come to be consumed my thoughts. Was he attacking her? Was this why he wanted to sit in on her sessions? Was he trying to keep her from talking? Did he somehow think a massage would make the bruises disappear? I wanted no part in his cover-up.

I could feel my face becoming hot, and I began to tremble as I tried to lay comforting hands on her. I asked more times than normal about the pressure and even if she wanted me to skip her legs. She said it was fine to continue but nothing else. I was hoping for an explanation, a sign that she needed help, tears, or something, since she *had* to know I could see this. But there was nothing.

I found myself glaring at her boyfriend angrily. He never even looked up. How smug he was, sitting over in the corner, knowing that I could see the bruises. Were they there last week? How could I have missed it? Were her reluctance to him coming into the room and her comment about jealousy subtle cries for help? There was no way I could ask because he was sitting *right there.*

He did have headphones on. Maybe I could whisper softly and she would tell me. But what could I say? *Is he beating you?* What would she say? Yes? Then what?

The room seemed small all of a sudden. I began to feel claustrophobic. I realized how unsafe my position was. This was stupider than the time I'd accepted a new male client and went to his house the very next day for a 7 pm appointment. How money hungry must I have been? At least then, I'd texted 5 people his address and where he worked. I'd called them right when I arrived and told them to call me immediately at the time it was supposed to be over. You can never be too safe, right?

When I undraped her back, there were even bruises on her sides. This guy was really doing a number on her. He'd left no part of her body untouched.

When the massage was over, I ran up front, trying to think of something I could do to help her. Maybe I'd write her a note on a small piece of paper and slip it to her. I could lock him out of the building, and she'd be safe until we could call the police. Maybe I could call the police now and they'd be here before they left. No, that wouldn't work. Then the door opened. He came out and closed the door behind him.

"Do you have a restroom in here?" he asked.

"Oh sure. It's right down the hall and to the left." *Perfect.* It was the only chance I'd have. I waited for him to close the bathroom door and stood right outside the treatment room. As soon as she opened the door, I gently pushed her back in and closed the door behind me. "Is everything okay?" I asked.

"What?" she asked, sounding confused.

"Is everything...*okay*?" I repeated, pointing to her legs. "He's in the restroom now." I whispered.

"Umm...yeah?" she asked like she wanted me to

elaborate.

"Are you sure?" I could here the bathroom door open. I looked at her, my eyes pleading with her to confirm what I knew was going on, but she was too afraid to say. Instead, she just stared at me quizzically. It was too late. I opened the door. "So I noticed some stiffness in your legs and back. Maybe next time we can focus more time there?" I played it off.

The three of us headed back up front. He paid and rebooked for the next week. The entire week, I researched what I should do as a massage therapist if I suspected abuse. Even if I reported it, she wasn't a child, disabled, or elderly. There was nothing I could do except try to convince her to get out of the situation and get help. There was no way I could speak with her in private while he was in the room. I thought about calling her, but I couldn't risk him hearing the conversation. That might make matters worse.

By the time the next appointment came, I was an emotional wreck and exhausted from thinking of all the things I could try to do or say. I'm not big into energy work, but I do believe in transference of energy. For the first time in a long time, I was nervous. I hadn't been this antsy since my first time working on a real client in student clinic. I tried to stay composed.

When they arrived, I figured he wanted to be in the room again. To my surprise, he was only dropping her off. I had mentally prepared myself for being trapped in the room with this abusive monster again but hadn't considered how I would approach the situation if she had the freedom to talk. I decided that we had an entire hour in private so I didn't need to rush this.

I didn't normally initiate conversation with clients, but if ever there was a need, this was it. When I entered the room, I began working on her neck and shoulders like normal. "I'm surprised he didn't want to stay again. Did he have to work?"

"No. He stays because an hour isn't long enough to go all the way home and come back. I guess he found something else to do today."

"Oh." I wasn't really sure what to say next. "Last week, I noticed you had a few bruises on your arms and legs. I hope the pressure was okay. Sometimes massage is good because it helps the blood circulate."

"Oh, yeah. Sorry about that. I bruise easily. I probably should have told you."

"Oh, it's okay. Lots of clients bruise easily. I try to be mindful of pressure if that's the case."

"No, the pressure is perfect. They're almost healed now, so it's no big deal."

I couldn't think of what to say next. I felt like there was a long, awkward pause. Maybe not for her because she was probably trying to relax and enjoy the little bit of freedom she had from the presence of her abuser.

I had tried being subtle but it wasn't working. Before long, the session would be over and he would be back. I needed her to know that this was a safe space for her. I needed her to understand that, if anything happened while she was home, she could call me and I would help in whatever way I could.

When I got to her arms and saw the bruises were worse, my heart sank. How long had she been living like this? She'd claimed she bruised easily but this was ridiculous. The number of bruises on her body was inexcusable. I've never been a victim of domestic abuse, so I never try to say what I would do if I were in the situation. I did know I would hate myself if something happened to her that could have been avoided. So I said something.

"These bruises seem to be worse than last time. Is everything okay? I tried asking last week, but I didn't want to put you on the spot, especially because he was here. This is a safe space. Is there anything I can do to help?" I was impressed that I was even able to go through the entire spiel, as nervous as I was.

She looked perplexed, like I was speaking a foreign language. She looked at her arms, smiled, and then laughed hysterically. "Oh my God!" At this point, she was laughing so hard she couldn't catch her breath. She began coughing through the laugh. I stepped back, confused, and offered her some water. She laughed and coughed "Yes!"

I stepped out of the room, unsure whether to be angry at her reaction or relieved. I headed to the mini fridge, grabbed a bottle of water, and then re-entered the treatment room.

She was sitting up on the table, holding the blanket with one hand to cover her breasts. The other hand was wiping tears from her eyes, and she was still laughing. I handed her the water, and she drank almost half the bottle before she stopped to regain her composure.

"You thought my boyfriend was beating me?" She laughed some more. "I'm a dancer! These bruises are from the pole! My boyfriend is going to think this is so funny."

I was both embarrassed and relieved at the same time. I can't recall which emotion was greater. For a week I had been in emotional turmoil over how to approach this client. It turned out she was just a stripper who didn't think to inform her therapist of her injuries from her job. My embarrassment shifted to anger. I'm not even sure if I hid it well.

I was mad that she wasn't considerate enough to explain her bruising. Mad that she didn't appreciate the care and compassion I was trying to show her. Even though I was wrong, she still could have been thankful for the gesture. Many women are abused and have no one to help them. I'm glad someone found humor in the situation because I sure didn't.

When the massage ended, her boyfriend was already waiting in the lobby to pick her up. He paid and rescheduled her next session. She came up the hall and began laughing as soon as she saw him.

"Babe, you'll never guess what she thought my bruises were from. She thought you were beating me!" She laughed.

Her boyfriend looked at me. I don't know if he was hurt or offended because I couldn't get myself to look him in the face. I focused on my computer to rebook her appointment, but I didn't hide my annoyance.

"I saw the bruises and wasn't sure. We see a lot of different clients on the table and most times, bruising like that is a sign of abuse." I stated as professionally as I could. The truth was I had never seen bruises that bad. I had never seen a client I suspected was being abused.

Fortunately, in my long career, I've never experienced another client who I suspected was being abused. If another person did come across my table, I believe I would do the same thing. I'd much rather risk embarrassment than live with myself knowing I didn't do everything I could to potentially save a life.

41

POOR GIRL

We are only privileged with the amount of information another person is willing to share. A lack of information forces us to piece together the story of another person's life, limited only by our own past experiences and selfish imagination. Intentions rarely matter. We are all guilty of judging and being judged.

There was nothing special about Poor Girl. She was an early twenty-something graduate student who was new to the spa. Her massage must have been a treat for the hard work she was putting in. I reviewed her new client form and could read her stuck-up tone all throughout.

Address: *The rich side of town*
Occupation: *Graduate Student in Amazing University*
Referred by: *Super Rich Fiancé*
Signature: *Super dramatic loops, rainbows, and sparkles*

The actual words were different, of course, but I heard her voice nonetheless.

I greeted Poor Girl after reviewing her new client form and forced my face to smile. She lifted her delicate hand to mine like it was too fragile to be shaken. I did so more out of habit than an attempt to be polite. She must have expected her belongings to be fetched and carried because when we arrived to the treatment room, she asked where they were.

"Oh, you didn't mean to leave them in the lobby?" I asked rhetorically.

She headed back to the front to retrieve her coat and out-of-season, mid-level designer handbag that I'm sure no one would dare to steal. She was in search of a new massage therapist. Her *rich fiancé* wanted her to not be so stressed while she finished her graduate school studies in a subject I can't quite remember. "He'll be paying for my weekly sessions." She made sure to flash her shiny ring as she waved her perfectly manicured hands obnoxiously about.

Poor Girl was the stereotypical person everyone assumed I came into contact with daily by working at a spa: rich snobs who talked down to you. Only the stereotype was wrong. Most of my regular clients treated me like a normal person. They cared about my studies and future career plans. But Poor Girl was the stereotype that I always said didn't exist. She talked down to everyone, never said thank you, and acted unimpressed with everything in the spa. Still, I kept my professionalism intact. I must have, since she scheduled every future session with me.

A few months into our boring sessions, Poor Girl

came in with four other women who were from out of town. They were sitting in the relaxation area, happily laughing and sipping glasses of champagne they'd brought with them to enjoy.

Poor Girl felt the need to introduce me to her family like we were friends of many years. I barely even knew her, since we'd never spoken during our sessions. I couldn't care less about her mother, her sisters, or the other woman who turned out to be her future mother-in-law. Good for her. I wasn't giving them massages, nor would I ever see them again.

They were here for a mini bridal shower. There were gift bags, champagne bottles, and small party favors. It seemed silly to me to have a shower at the spa when they could have easily done the gift-giving at home and just come here for the massage.

I learned one glass of champagne made Poor Girl chatty. I suffered through the entire massage hearing about her perfect fiancé and how he was the one who'd encouraged her to get frequent massage. In fact, he was so adamant that she *take care of herself* that he paid for all of them. She must have forgotten she'd shared that information the first day we'd met.

There was something about her that made me hate every word that escaped her mouth. Everything I had in life, I'd worked hard to obtain. I couldn't afford a massage because it would cost me three hours worth of pay, which needed to go toward my rent. Trading sessions wasn't free or reliable. If a client wanted in during the time I was scheduled, I got *bumped* for a full paying client. Here she was, living my dream of weekly massages, graduate school, and a fiancé who spoiled her to no end. Life was unfair. She would never know a life of struggle and would go on to live her life happily ever after.

Yet, still, I maintained my professional composure. I smiled and congratulated her. I gave her another great massage. I wished her luck and figured I'd see her when she changed her name…

TICKLED PINK

Over the years, I've lost count of the number people I've touched. The ones who've managed to occupy a permanent residence in my memory are those who have touched me back in one way or another.

Mr. Pink was booked monthly appointments but never with the same massage therapist. While none of us questioned why, I think we all held out hope that we would each break the cycle and become his requested therapist. But after the appointments, no therapist was ever offended by the fact that he bounced around from room to room, never choosing a favorite among us. We each very much preferred it that way.

Mr. Pink eventually landed on my table a few months after I started working at a massage practice located in an old beat-up office building. His client file was one of the thickest I had ever seen. It struck me as odd that the only area of concern was his neck, yet the information the therapists shared seemed to span the length of the page.

I skimmed through the first three entries, saw the similarities, and decided that was all the information I needed. Okay, I get it. Light pressure, don't talk, let him lie on his side and spend a little more time on the neck. Too easy.

When I met Mr. Pink, I didn't initially pick up on the creepy vibe. I greeted him with confidence, firmly shook his dainty hand, and led the way back to the treatment room. He walked back to the room in a way that looked more like a glide. His movements were so graceful, it was almost beautiful to watch.

With his file in hand, I reviewed his past appointments with him.

"So it looks like your past few visits, you needed extra time on your neck and preferred light pressure?" I asked for confirmation.

"Correct." He stared at me with a blank expression.

"Okay. And you prefer side lying? Is this due to an injury or discomfort?"

"Preference." Another blank stare.

"Can we begin with you face-up? It's much easier and more effective to work on your neck while your face up than on your side."

"No." He gave no hint of agitation, just replied in a matter-of-fact tone.

"No problem. I can adjust," I conceded. He was the client, and it was his session. His comfort and preference were what mattered.

I entered the room prepared to work on this client

like any other. He laid on the table, cradling one of the pillows.

"Are you comfortable?"

"Can we not speak please?"

"No problem." That simple request felt like a gut punch. I tried not to take it personally, as it was possible he may have had negative experiences with past therapists who may have been overly chatty. I pushed the cold request to the back of my mind and began with the massage.

"I asked for light pressure," he snapped.

"Do you need me to go lighter?" I asked while adjusting the pressure of my hands.

"Lighter please, I will let you know when it's light enough." The statement seemed strange. Most people speak up when the pressure is too much to handle, but this was different. "Lighter please. A bit more. There. Thank you."

In the thousands of massages I've given in my entire career, the massage I gave Mr. Pink was by far the hardest on me physically. "There" was literally just light enough for the pads of my fingertips to ever so gently graze the surface of his skin. There was no need for oil or massage cream.

Interestingly enough, my first thought was never that he might have some sick fetish or twisted sociopathic desire to take a professional massage therapist to their breaking point. Those possibilities were introduced to me immediately after I left the room and discussed the massage with other therapists who had worked on him before.

Each of us shared a similar experience with him. A feather light touch, focus on his neck, no talking, and letting him lie on his side. Only after the massage did I understand the need to write a full page worth of text. Recalling my entire session.

Do not talk at all. VERY, VERY, VERY LIGHT PRESSURE. Wants focus on neck. Use a feather's worth of pressure. He will tell you when it's light enough. Do not ask questions. Do not use your entire hand. Light fingertip touch. Prefers side-lying. Will not speak. Do not use lotion. Light Touch Only.

Only after the massage did I take a bit more time to read the entirety of his client file. Every therapist in the past tried to warn the next. No therapist's name appeared in his chart twice.

The high employee turnover allowed for him to float effortlessly between new therapists, leaving us to come up with our own reasons for why he needed that type of work. I still refuse to believe his intentions were impure. It's best to believe people are genuinely in need of the things they request when you are faced with clients like Mr. Pink.

FAQ: "SO HOW DID YOU GET INTO THIS?"

Some people feel the need to make small talk in the massage room. Maybe they feel a little nervous, or maybe they don't like silence. Either way, there were very few original questions. In fact, I'd heard some of them a hundred times. Like, "So how did you get into this?" which I always answered with this story:

Another therapist and I were giving a couple's massage to these two ladies who were having a spa day. My client asked, "How'd you guys get into this?' I responded with my usual story of how I'd just tripped and fell into the industry. It was either going to be culinary arts or massage. I couldn't imagine being a sous chef, so massage school won out.

The other therapist, Tracy, replied, "Well the first time I got a massage, I loved how it felt, so I went to school for it."

Tracy's client said, "That's funny. My gynecologist said the same thing!"

This funny story always helped break the ice with nervous clients.

But some frequently asked questions didn't allow for a humorous answer. Like "Do you have a church home?" It was a common question, but one particular client made it memorable.

FAQ: "DO YOU HAVE A CHURCH HOME?"

If the lights weren't dim and his eyes were open, I may not have been able to mask my annoyance with this question. But he was a paying client, so I turned on the charm, even though I had been asked this question many times and I had always felt uncomfortable answering it. Someone should tell clients there are certain topics that are off-limits. Politics, sexual orientation, and religion are the top three.

It's easy to think you just won't answer or you'll simply change the subject until you're in the situation. Trapped inside a room with a pastor. Sometimes it's just easier to say what I did: "I'm still looking." In truth, I wasn't actively looking for a church home. It was not a priority for me at the time. Anytime a body on the table would ask, I always gave the same answer.

Most people took the hint and recognized the response to be a brush-off. Some would offer the name of their church, extend an invitation, and let that be the end of it. Not the pastor. He was either the most clueless person in existence or the most aggressive Christian salesman in America. Forty minutes of his first 60-minute massage session was spent with me dodging religious probes. By the end, I had gained a new regular client and he had a new church attendee. We both won.

Our client-therapist relationship lasted almost a year, starting at a spa and continuing well into my private mobile practice. Over the course of our relationship, our conversations turned personal. My guess is this happens with clients where the relationship exists beyond the confines of the treatment room. I can't be certain, since this was the first and last time it happened for me.

I arrived for what would become our last session, only neither of us knew it. I showed up at my usual time, ten minutes early, to allow myself time to set up. He answered the door in his robe. We politely greeted each other, and I set up in my usual spot. He did his usual. He offered to help, which I declined. He offered a beverage, which I declined. I excused myself to wash my hands down the hall to allow him time to disrobe and get on the table.

Often, I extended the amount of time necessary to wash my hands. I learned this lesson the hard way. I had accidentally walked in on enough half-naked bodies over the years to know better than to return too soon.

I admired the fake plastic flowers in the pastor's

guest bathroom. I had seen those flowers plenty of times, but this was my routine. I checked my hair and pulled it back tight. I ran my hands under the warm water for a few seconds then wrapped them tightly in my personal hand towel, hoping they would be warm upon first touch. I cracked the door and asked loudly, "You all set?" He confirmed that he was ready.

I returned to his open living room and began adjusting the sheet and blanket that had gotten tangled in the process of him getting on the table. My client was well over 500lbs. I still hadn't gotten around to purchasing a set of sheets larger than twin size to accommodate his larger frame. If not for the queen size blanket, I doubt the sheets alone would have been enough to protect the privacy my client deserved. With the sheet and blanket neatly adjusted, I began. My hands were cold and he shuddered.

"Can I ask you a question?"

"Sure."

"The first time you came to my church, was the guy you brought your boyfriend?"

"No, he was just a friend." The question caught me off guard. I wasn't sure how to answer. The man in question was a person I had dated off and on for years. I felt guilty admitting that to my pastor. We weren't exclusive, so I felt my response was as honest as I was willing to share.

"Did you know my first massage was with you?"

"Really?" The memory of our first session was still vivid in my mind because of the aggressive religious interrogation.

"Yeah. I always wanted to try one but I was scared."

"Of what?" I genuinely chuckled. "Well I guess you guys are in a vulnerable position. We could kill you on the table with one move." We laughed.

"Honestly, that I'd break the table."

"Oh, these tables are sturdier than they look and mine ain't cheap." I smiled, impressed with myself that I was able to quickly recover from what would only be the beginning of a 90-minute awkward situation. I relied on humor to navigate me through many situations. This happened to be one.

"Yeah, but I didn't know what to expect. Somebody seeing me. Even with women, personally, I've always been nervous. You know, women, they find out I'm a pastor and they get uncomfortable, too. They start pretending to be saints." As I listened, my stomach began to turn, and I could feel the pulse in my fingertips. Was I exposed? "But you were just sweet. You talked to me like a normal person. I haven't even dated anyone in years because I just don't want to be disappointed. I just know she's gonna look at me and be disgusted because I'm so…BIG!"

I pushed my own thoughts aside as I struggled to massage his thighs, which were wider than my waist.

"But if she likes you, she won't care. In fact, I don't date small guys. I like big guys. I'm tiny myself. I need a guy big enough where I don't question whether I can whoop his ass. If I even *think* I can give him some go, he's not my type." I chuckled. "I'm like a tiny Chihuahua. Lots of bark and no bite. So if we're ever in public and I get us into some mess, I need people to look at my guy and think twice before they make a move." He belted out a hearty laugh and smiled.

My comments were innocent but not entirely true. In fact, the man I'd brought with me to church was 6 feet even and barely weighed 180 pounds. While I preferred a muscular build, my heart did not discriminate.

"Have you ever considered modeling?"

The questions were coming from left field. Most of our conversations were about scripture, weekend plans, and business goals. This was out of character. "Um, no. I'm too shy for that." I never saw myself as someone attractive enough to be a model. Even if I had, I'd always been too shy for public adoration. I never knew how to take a compliment, so modeling would never be for me.

"Really? I could see you modeling on a perm box or something."

I'd never laughed harder in a session. I supposed it was a compliment but not one I had heard before. He fell silent while I envisioned my face on the side of a box of relaxers. What brand would it be? Olive Oil? Motions?

For the first time ever, he was quiet for the remainder of the session. During the silence, I realized too late that my attempt at delivering a sympathetic confidence booster by saying I liked big guys could be mistaken for flirtation. Lucky for me, the conversation stopped before I could say anything more. The massage was completed without another word spoken. There was nothing but his labored breathing over the sound of my favorite classical piano music being played on my portable radio.

I excused myself to wash my hands and mentally kicked myself for such a poor choice of conversation. I looked at myself in the mirror and mouthed *YOU IDIOT! UGH! WHY WOULD YOU SAY THAT! STUPID! STUPID! STUPID!*

If you ever wondered whether scrubbing your hands furiously could somehow defy all odds and allow you to travel back in time to get a redo, it's been confirmed. It doesn't. I cracked the door open. "All dressed?"

"I'm good."

Normally, he disappeared into his bedroom to redress in private while I cleared and packed my table and belongings. Instead, he sat comfortably on the couch in a loosely tied robe and offered me a bottle of water.

"No thanks," I said, slightly exhausted from the 90-minute session I had just given.

"How much is it today?"

"$145, as usual." I smiled, avoiding eye contact as I zipped my bag and headed toward the door.

"If you don't have another client later, maybe we

can get some lunch?"

"Oh, I actually do," I lied. "It's across town, so I have to get going."

"Don't you eat in between? At least let me get you some water, some snacks…something." He seemed to be expressing genuine concern.

"I'm good." I smiled. "Will you need change?" I asked, drawing attention to the fact that he still hadn't paid me.

"No, no. Let me go grab my wallet." He disappeared into his bedroom and returned shortly with two $100 bills.

"Oh, thank you. You sure you don't need change?" I smiled uncomfortably. He'd tipped before, maybe $15 or $20 but never $55.

"Nah, nah. That's yours. Thank you. Two weeks?"

"Sure. Send me a text." I turned and headed out the door.

Over the next two weeks, his texts made it more obvious that my comments had been misinterpreted. He requested dates, dinners, and to know the reason I hadn't been at church. The messages finally stopped 10 minutes after I didn't show up for his next scheduled appointment.

A line had been crossed due to a thoughtless comment that slipped out of my mouth. From then on, I made it a point to never make that mistake again. I felt terrible not responding and no showing, but what was I going to say? How could I recover? I wasn't interested in more and couldn't risk inserting my foot in my mouth again. I took the coward's way out.

FAQ: "DO YOUR HANDS EVER HURT?"

The massage space can be one of extreme vulnerability. Clients trust us with all of their insecurities, pain, and sometimes emotions. Because of that, professional boundaries sometimes become blurry the closer two people become.

While I joked with the pastor about clients being in a vulnerable position, practically naked on a table with a stranger who could probably kill them with one touch, the amount of times I've felt vulnerable were too many to count. The sexual propositions never ended. Looking back, I can admit it was me who put myself in those questionable and sometimes dangerous situations. Before I relied on humor, I leveraged the power of a smile. Blame it on youth, ignorance, or just plain stupidity, I used my not-so-innocent smile to guide the wrong clients right to my table.

I met a car salesman one day during an aggressive self-marketing campaign. One day, out of the blue, I gathered up my brochures, business cards, and massage table and headed straight to a luxury car dealership. My ego was quickly deflated when the manager refused to let me set up my table, but he told me I could leave my business cards. I was sure my cards would find their new home in a trash bin the moment I turned my back to leave.

On my way out the door, a salesman approached me. He'd overheard my failed attempt to pitch my services. He was another unicorn who was pleased to see a black massage therapist in real life.

"So you really do massage? There are black massage therapists?"

"Yes. There are a few of us. I've been licensed for three years." BAM! I shot him that smile.

"Oh? Where do you work?" He grinned back and bit his lower lip. Why do men do that?

"For myself. I do in-home and office massage."

"So you do outcall?"

"That's another way of saying it, I guess."

"So when are you gonna come to my house? I get massages all the time." He laughed in a way that that let me know it wasn't a serious question. Only I was willing to call his bluff.

"When you call to book your appointment." BAM! Another smile.

"How much?"

"$120."

"Dang! For a massage?"

"Yes," I said without breaking eye contact. I stated my prices with confidence. "You sell luxury cars, why can't I sell luxury massage?" I handed him a card and walked out the door.

That did the trick because within an hour he sent me a text.

> *- When can you come by?*
> *When you book your appointment —*
> *- That's what I'm trying to do*
> *I have availability tomorrow. What time would you prefer? —*
> *- 7 pm*
> *That's pretty late. I take my last appointment at 5 for safety reasons —*
> *- I get off at 5. It's not like you don't know where I work*
> *Good point. Send your address. I'll be there around 6:45 —*

The next day, I felt very nervous leading up to the massage. He was the first client I'd agreed to do a house call for without having a prior relationship, nor was he referred to me by someone I knew.

I talked things over with a few close friends. Each expressed genuine concern for me going to a man's house I didn't know. I eased their concern by promising to forward them his address and photo and calling the moment I arrived. I made sure to sound as confident as possible and not allow my fear to be revealed in my voice. I must have succeeded because none of my friends put up much more of a fight.

I packed up my truck and placed his address in my navigation system. It would take approximately 35 minutes to arrive. He lived in a suburb of the main city. As I got closer, I was surprised to find he lived in an apartment and not a house. Not that it mattered, but most of my clients lived in what I called rich people houses. His mediocre lifestyle didn't match my expectations.

When I arrived, I knocked, waited a bit, and then rang the doorbell. I double-checked my phone to make sure I had the correct address. I did. I squatted down to throw the strap of the bag that held my table over my shoulder and headed back to my car.

Once back in my car, I called his number. It only took two rings.

"Hello?"

"Hi, it's Kamillya. We had a massage scheduled tonight. I'm here at your place and there's no answer."

"Oh, you said 7. My bad, I was in the shower. Give me a few minutes."

I waited anxiously in the car until I saw the light appear when he opened the front door. He stood at about 6'1", with no shirt and long basketball shorts. I gathered my table and portable radio and headed to the door.

"Oh you wasn't playing." He laughed and offered to help carry the table. I declined.

"Yes. This is my table. How did you think you were getting a massage?"

"I don't know. I never had one on a table before."

I stupidly ignored this comment and didn't ask the question that I should have. *I thought you said you get massages all the time?* Future Kamillya would have asked. Future Kamillya would not have put herself in this position in the first place. Future Kamillya needed to learn this hard lesson in order to make better-informed decisions and not bait clients through flirtation and that damned smile.

Setting up the table was awkward to say the least. His townhouse apartment housed large furniture, so finding a place to fit my table was a challenge. We settled on the entryway right by the front door. It was barely wide enough to fit between the wall and kitchen bar, but I made do. Sometimes being very thin has its benefits. He watched me set up my table and made no effort to break his gaze.

"Where's the restroom?"

"Just around the corner and straight back."

"Okay, I'm going to go wash my hands. You can undress and climb between these two sheets. Go ahead and start face down for me with your face in this hole here." I didn't normally start my clients face down, but something about this guy didn't feel right. Future Kamillya learned to trust her gut the hard way.

I was surprised by the cleanliness of his bathroom. Most men his age didn't keep their home this tidy. He was mid-20s, and judging by the furniture and décor, he was doing quite well for himself. Maybe he could be a good regular client, after all. I may have found a diamond in the rough. After washing my hands and staring at myself for a while in the bathroom mirror, I finally cracked the door.

"All set?"

"Yeah." I could hear that his voice was muffled by the face cradle.

When I returned to the entryway, he was lying on top of the blanket, still in his shorts and socks. It was clear he'd never had a professional massage. I didn't want to embarrass him, so I didn't draw any unnecessary attention. Instead, I simply asked, "Are you comfortable?"

"Mmmhmm."

"So are there any areas that you need me to focus on?" I was so out of my element that I hadn't even done a proper intake prior to him getting on my table. Future Kamillya would always do a proper intake before beginning any massage.

"Yeah, my back," he said, reaching his arms around to touch his lower back.

"Okay, I'll spend some extra time there on your lower back. Feel free to speak up if the pressure is too much."

"I like deep. You can't hurt me, so go as deep as you want."

"Do you just want me to focus on upper body since you left your shorts and socks on?" The words sounded purely professional coming out of my mouth. But I could only hear what I wanted. Future Kamillya would always be mindful of how a client could interpret her words.

"Oh, I didn't know. You want me to take them off?"

"No. If this is comfortable for you, I can just work around them."

As I worked on his back, I noticed him flinching and recoiling at the pressure, so I backed off. He began sharing stories of his two children and how he only got to see them a few times a month. At the time, I didn't have children and couldn't understand the level of emotion that began pouring out of him. He went on about how the mother of his children had fought to take custody and made him pay more than he could afford in child support.

I listened without judgment but found myself wondering what his children looked like. I imagined them running up and down the stairs, playing, and enjoying time with their father like I used to as a child.

My thoughts were interrupted when he abruptly changed the subject.

"Hey, what are you doing after this?"

"Nothing planned. Just home and sleep. I have a client early in the morning."

"You should go out with me and some of my boys tonight. We're gonna pregame here and probably hit up some clubs later."

"No. I have an early appointment. Plus, I don't go out with clients."

"Dang, I'm just a client? We can't be friends?"

"I prefer money over friends."

"Dang. Well you should let me massage you after you finish. I give massages all the time. I'm told I'm pretty good."

"No thanks. I'm sure what you do is not a professional massage. Plus, people who don't do this professionally usually can't last more than five minutes tops. I'd rather get a real massage." Still, hearing my own words, they sounded innocent and professional. Future Kamillya would disagree.

"Trust me, I can last longer than five minutes."

I'm certain I was naïve to the meaning of his comment. That's the story I'm sticking to.

The massage was halfway over, and it was time for him to turn. Since he'd left his shorts on, it was an easy process. When clients are under the sheets, I have to lean into the side table to secure the top sheet and blanket so they don't pull it with them when they turn. I needed to reach over them and lift the linens on the far side of the table so they never became exposed. He wasn't under the sheets, so I said, "Alright. It's time for you to turn over. Slide down just a bit so your head is on the table and not in the face rest."

He did as instructed and cupped his hands to shield his erection. I pretended not to notice. It wasn't the first and wouldn't be the last time this had happened. I decided to begin working on his neck and shoulders, hoping it would subside and I could move on to work his arms later. I began talking to him to ease any embarrassment he may have had.

"So how long have you been working at the luxury dealership?"

"A few months. A friend of mine helped me get it. His dad owns the dealership. That's who I'm hanging out with tonight. You sure you don't want to go? He's supposed to be bringing some drinks by later tonight."

"I don't drink," I lied. It was much easier than navigating around another advance.

"Oh. So you're a good girl? We might have to change that."

I was never good in these situations. Even off the table, I didn't handle overt flirtation well. I'm the first to admit that my level of social awkwardness hits a ten when faced with responding to advances, whether I'm interested or not. I was not interested in him and was uncertain how to navigate my way out. So I laughed and smiled. Damn that stupid smile.

I finished his neck and shoulders and stood to begin working on one of his hands.

"Your hands are soft," he said as he watched my hands work. I always hated when clients watched me massage them. There's something strange about it.

"Thank you." I smiled again. Damn it.

"You got a man?"

"No." *Why didn't I say yes?*

"That's a shame. I'm sure if you did, he'd be trying to get massages every day."

"And he would fail. This is work. I wouldn't want

to come home and work after massaging people all day. I hope whoever I end up with will understand that."

"See, if I was your man, I'd massage you every day. I'd rub your feet because you'd been standing all day. Rub your back and make sure you felt good every day." He watched me massage him as I moved to the other side of the table and began working on his other hand. "Do your hands ever get tired?"

He reached down in his shorts for what I hoped would be a quick adjustment. Instead he lowered his shorts and revealed himself to me right there on my table and pulled my wrist to touch him. I jerked away without a word. I ran to lock myself in the bathroom. *Damn, why didn't I run out the front door?* Future Kamillya would have run out the front door.

I locked the bathroom door behind me, terrified that he might try to come inside. I had no phone and nothing to defend myself with if something else were to happen. I searched the bathroom for something, anything I could use as a weapon. There was nothing. Damn his pristine bathroom.

I could hear him scramble off the table. Maybe I'd scared him as much as he'd scared me.

"What you doing? Ain't nobody gone do nothing to you. You ain't gotta hide in the bathroom. My bad, dang."

I sat on the toilet until I could control my breathing and tried to figure out how I was going to escape. *If I leave the bathroom will he grab me? Will I collect my things or make a run for the door? Should I scream for help? Should I call the police?*

"Girl, come get your stuff. I'm not about to do nothing to you."

Reluctantly, I unlocked the door and slowly stepped out. I could barely hear his apologies due to the blood that rushed to my head and clouded my hearing. My face felt hot. I was angry with him and myself for not putting an end to the session sooner.

I snatched off the sheets and quickly collapsed the table. My hands fumbled with the bag until I finally gave up and carried my bare table outside with the sheets and bag all balled in one. My phone buzzed on the bar stool, reminding me it was there. I stepped back into the apartment and retrieved it. Too afraid to answer, I sent the call to voicemail. It was my friend making sure I was okay. The phone buzzed again. And again.

I answered hastily, "Hey. I'm good. Just now leaving. I'll call you from the car." I hung up without waiting for a reply. I shut the door behind me, leaving my portable radio and favorite massage music CD. Maybe he still has it, or maybe it's in the trash. Future Kamillya couldn't care less about a lost CD and radio.

To answer his question honestly, yes my hands do get tired. Though I never understood why people ask this question. I sometimes wonder what would happen if I said, "Yes, they're actually tired right now." Would my client let me take a break? After this experience, I gave my hands a month-long break.

THAT GUY

____

The first time I worked on That Guy, he was only in for a 30-minute appointment. I knew from the moment I met him in the lobby that he wasn't my ideal client. He was rude and on his cell phone when I came out to greet him. I stood off to the side, within eyesight, waiting patiently so I wouldn't interrupt. He spoke loudly and used offensive language that caught the attention of the other waiting clients. So their experience wouldn't be affected, I walked up to him and smiled so he would know I was ready to take him back.

When clients are on their phones, it's always awkward. You don't want to be impolite and interrupt, but you also need to hurry them along so they don't lose valuable time on the table or cause you to fall behind on your schedule.

That Guy simply looked at me and stood. He didn't smile back, shake my hand, or end his call. The walk to the room was just as uncomfortable. He spoke loudly although I whispered for him to follow behind me. Most clients realize when you enter a dimly lit area or the other person is whispering that they should whisper, too. The fact that other treatment doors were closed should have been a sign that other services were in session and silence was appreciated. But That Guy didn't take the hints. He just went on with the same harsh tone and language as when I met him.

We arrived at my room, where he spent another two minutes wrapping up his call. Two minutes in the massage world is a very long time, especially when the treatment is only 30 minutes and there are clients on the schedule right afterward. When he finally finished his call, I began the interview. I asked what areas he needed focus on, hoping he wouldn't ask for a full body. Of course, he wanted a full body massage.

I informed him that it would not be beneficial for him to receive a full body treatment within 30 minutes and that the best we could do would be either upper or lower body. Visibly annoyed, he opted for the upper body. He commanded that I just wait outside the door because he would undress quickly and yell when he was ready.

I didn't oblige. Instead, I went to the break room, washed my hands, and took many deep breaths before returning to the room with the rude, demanding, and offensive client. When I returned, I tapped gently on the door, cracked it open slightly, and said, "All set?"

"I shouted for you to come in!" he barked as I

entered the room. I informed him that I'd needed to wash my hands prior to beginning his session and apologized for not returning fast enough. I assured him he'd get his full time and there was no need to worry.

There he was, about 6'5" long on the table, with only the top sheet covering him from the waist down. I noticed the top blanket thrown in the corner of the room on the floor. Apparently he was too hot for the blanket and took it upon himself to get more comfortable.

The tension in the room made it hard for me to breathe. The negative energy radiating from this client made it very hard to find a good flow. Then something strange happened.

Out of nowhere, That Guy began to speak. He talked to me like I was one of the guys he'd known for years, sharing tales of business travel and sexual exploits along the way. He spoke about the many women he met and how they weren't any good because they were just eyeing him for his money.

About halfway through, I asked him to turn over so I could spend the rest of the time on his back. My hope was that the one-sided conversation would finally end so I could put my hands on autopilot and allow my mind to escape to a far-off place and forget where I was. No such luck.

He spent the remaining time talking about how he'd only come here because *some girl* had purchased the gift certificate for him. She'd told him he was too stressed and needed to relax. Poor girl and poor me.

By the time the session finally ended, I'd learned of his travels all over the world and the many beautiful women that he'd met. I'd learned about his coworkers and how unlucky they were to be married because they missed out on all the fun. Except for John and James, who didn't care and still had their fun, too.

I left the room relieved that it was over and he'd only been there on a gift certificate. Usually these were one-time clients I would never see again. I met him outside the room with a cold bottle of spring water, thanked him for coming, and led him back up front. I returned to my room to find a $40 tip, which I believed I'd earned.

That Guy turned into a regularly irregular client who I very much hated. I dreaded seeing his name on my appointment book. Maybe I should have spoke up instead of responding with the polite "Uh huh" or "That sounds interesting." But the first time I figured it was only 30 minutes, why make the situation worse? His next appointment was a few months later, and he wanted a full 60 minutes. I expected it to be torture.

I was never a believer in all that energy talk that some therapists subscribed to, but when you're desperate, you'll look for any form of help. I asked for advice on what to do before going back into the room with That Guy. Before I go into the recommendations, let me tell you why I continued with the sessions.

When you work for a spa or any other employee-based position, if you're going to turn down a request, many times you need a really good reason. Remember the story of the unicorn: I had been fired in the past for making a complaint about a situation. The spa was the next place I worked after being fired from the chiropractic office, and let's just say the past experience stuck with me.

The biggest difference between the two workplaces was the staff support. I feared taking my concerns to the owner, however the other massage therapists on staff offered a mountain of advice. They told me to ground myself, change the subject, block his energy, or directly tell him to stop.

I continued on with the next session feeling better equipped to handle him. Once again, he was on his phone. This time, at least I received a nod when he saw me heading up the hall. He stood and began heading toward me before I reached the lobby. I turned around and headed to the treatment room with him following behind me on the phone. By the time we arrived in the treatment room, he had at least ended his conversation. I asked what areas needed attention, and he said, "Just do the same thing you did last time." It had been months since I'd last seen him, and that had only been a 30-minute treatment. Even if I did remember the session, it wouldn't be the same since this one was longer.

I'm not sure how most massage therapists operate, but I have a fall-back routine. Unless the client has specific issues or our bodies are really in alignment with one another, I always have a routine that I can throw my hands into autopilot, simply tune out, and perform. I had been following the routine for so long that it was timed down to the last minute or so of the massage. This ability came in very handy while working in a spa, where most people just want to relax. Only with That Guy, I couldn't get into my zone.

Once again, I entered the room to him grumbling about me taking too long to come back. My blanket was tossed again on the floor in the corner. All the grounding work I'd done leading up to coming into the room with a clear head did me no good. I proceeded with the massage anyway.

The standard sized massage tables do nothing for those who do not fall within average size, both in length and width. Clients who are wider than average may not be able to lie comfortably with their arms at their sides. Clients who are very tall will probably have their feet stick out past the edge of the table. Lucky for That Guy, I was very thin and even in the tiny room, I was able to make my way around the end of the table without my body brushing against his feet.

Barely 10 minutes into the massage, the speaking began. He shared tales of his most recent travels and experiences abroad, ignoring the fact that he was speaking to a woman. Maybe my feelings didn't matter. I could never get why some people needed to fill silence with the sound of their own voice, never noticing that the other person is not reciprocating. I used to always feel like clients only speak if they think we are friends or just can't relax. Whenever a client would ask, I would openly tell them they shouldn't feel obligated to talk. My feelings would never be hurt. A successful conversation is when both parties are engaged and contributing equally. Maybe he missed the memo.

By the time the session was over, I was more exhausted from his stories than from the actual session. I met him back outside the room with a bottle of water, smiled, thanked him for coming, and gestured for him to head to the front and pay. I re-entered the room to find a $5 tip. I hoped it was a sign that he was displeased and would never come again. I checked my schedule after he left, and he was not there. I felt relieved.

Six months passed before I saw That Guy again. When he scheduled, he couldn't remember my name but wanted to make sure he was scheduled with *the black girl*. The receptionist didn't act like she didn't know who he was referring to, but for some reason, made it a point to let me know that's how he requested me. Twice he had come to me and now twice he'd requested me and didn't remember my name. I felt small, like I was beneath him and less than a person. Maybe it wasn't his intention, but it's how I felt.

The appointment was now for 90 minutes, and I

couldn't imagine what I would do. The past two sessions, I couldn't seem to throw my hands into autopilot. I was very aware of every stroke, every word, and every move that took place during his sessions.

To prepare myself for this session, I made certain to remove the top blanket, neatly folding and storing it beneath the massage table. I wanted to make sure his session began and ended better than the last two. Prior to greeting him in the lobby, I washed my hands and planned to stand and wait outside the door.

When I greeted That Guy in the lobby, he was not on his phone. Instead, he was sitting quietly, his eyes closed, and his attire was very casual compared to how he'd dressed in the past. "Are you ready to head back?" I said softly so as not to abruptly jolt him from his relaxed state. He opened his eyes and stood without a word. For the first time, other clients in session did not have to overhear his phone conversation in the hall. When we entered the room, I asked where he needed focus, and he requested the same as last time. I'd expected as much.

I stood outside the door and waited for him to shout that he was ready. About three minutes later, I still heard nothing. I knocked softly and cracked the door. "All set?"

"Mmmhmm," he grumbled.

I entered the room with lead feet and fought myself not to watch the clock. An hour and a half isn't particularly long, but it can feel like an eternity when you're with a client you don't like. He said he was cold. I retrieved the blanket from under the table and stretched it across his body. I asked if he had traveled this week. He requested that we not speak this session.

I sat on my stool behind his head to begin the session. He inhaled deeply and exhaled through a wide open mouth. My nose caught a hint of stale alcohol on his breath. He was hung over. His misery would finally be the gift I needed to make it through the long session.

Just as I began to tune out and get into my zone, he spoke. He went on about the night he'd had with the guys at a bachelor party. Women were everywhere, doing everything. Having worked on him a few times before, I had already built up a wall to block out the mental images he felt so comfortable sharing. I gave no sign that I was interested in his tales.

Maybe he needed me to be his sounding board. To share the things he couldn't share so freely anywhere else. Once the treatment room door closed, many clients have been known to share some of their most deep, dark secrets without the therapist ever needing to pry. What was it about lying on the table that just makes people open up? I never asked.

We neared the end of the massage and the details became more and more graphic. I found it unbelievable that at no point did he ever consider that I might not want to hear these things. Then the massage was over. I met him outside the treatment room with a bottle of water, smiled, and gestured him to the front to check out. Later that day, I checked my schedule and That Guy was scheduled for a couples massage two weeks out.

I can't even lie. I was curious who this woman could be. Probably some brainless piece of arm candy who was only with him for the money. This man complained every chance he could about the women he ran into.

The next two weeks flew by and I didn't give his appointment too much thought. Most times, clients are silent during a couple's massage, and I expected his to be the same.

The day of his massage, I ran into a client I knew in the lobby: Poor Girl. I hadn't seen her in some weeks since our last session and was surprised to see her in the spa. She wasn't booked with me, so I felt a bit cheated on.

I greeted her with a fake "Hi, it's good to see you. How was the wedding?" I didn't really care about her wedding, but it was either that or make her feel bad for not scheduling her appointment with me. Not only was her life perfect, she was now cheating on me with another therapist in the spa.

"It was perfect. We just got back from a week in Europe for our honeymoon. It was magical." Who says *magical?* How phony. "Am I booked with you today?"

"I don't think so. I've got a regular client today, so

I don't think I'll be able to take you now. My next hour is free though if you're just walking in."

"No, my husband booked us a couple's massage. He's just parking the car."

A huge grin spread across my face. I didn't even feel guilty. There was so much that I knew about That Guy she had just married that made up for all the times she was rude and inconsiderate. All the times she talked around me or made me feel small disappeared from my mind.

When That Guy walked through the door, I greeted him as usual. The other therapist met me in the lobby and introduced herself to Poor Girl…or now Mrs. Guy. Poor Girl looked at me, then back at her husband and playfully shouted, "You stole my therapist!" I just smiled.

"Oh you see her, too? I didn't know. If you want her, we can trade."

"It's fine. I see her every week. You can have her today."

They spoke around me like I was a toy instead of a person. That wasn't surprising, since my past experiences with them were pretty much the same.

By the time we made it back to the couple's room, the fact that I had been seeing his wife over the past year finally clicked. The memories of our past conversations would not go over so well if she knew what he'd shared. For the first time ever, my entire massage with That Guy was in silence. I could turn off my brain and throw my hands in autopilot like I had been dreaming of doing from the day we'd met. In one session, I was able to silence an obscene talker and overcome the envy I was feeling toward the other client in the room.

Her life was no more perfect than my own. I was a struggling college student with two jobs, mounting debt, and no savings, but I could honestly say I would never trade my life for hers. It was the last time I saw either of those clients again. They both shook my hand and tipped very handsomely after the couple's massage.

I've always been curious if he was more embarrassed and worried than he needed to be. I believe he either stopped paying for her to receive massages, or maybe they found a new spa. Whatever the reason, they both stopped coming to me. I wish them a happy ending. I certainly had mine.

95

THE LONG APOLOGY

As a black massage therapist working in a predominately white industry, these questions come up a lot. "Do you ever get people who don't want you to massage them because you're black?" "When people see that you are giving them the massage, do they ever request someone else?" "Has anyone ever said anything racist to you in the room?" I never claim to speak for other therapists, but I expect each of us has had our own experiences.

Did I ever have anyone not want me to give them a massage because I am black? If they didn't, they never made me aware of it. I suspect if it ever was the case, clients just suffered through the session in miserable silence. Their worst nightmare of being trapped in a room with a black person touching all over them was now coming true.

I'm certain black males have it harder than black women. I've seen the fear cross the face of many clients. I've known people to comfortably receive a massage from a white male, but they couldn't bear to be touched by a black one. Those clients are few and far between, but I've witnessed it.

When people saw that I was the one giving them the massage, did they ever request someone else? If they did, I was never made aware of it. I'm not sure any person would openly admit that was the reason they didn't want me as a therapist. I've been discriminated against for being small, though. Clients assumed I wouldn't be able to give enough pressure because I didn't look strong enough. I've had that happen many times, but never because I'm black…at least not that I'm aware of.

Has a client ever said anything racist to me in the room? Yes. Many times. Clients have a tendency to think that, because they're a regular and tip generously, we're friends. And friends can tell *jokes*. And *jokes* aren't offensive. But they are. When you're young and lack experience dealing with certain situations, you don't have the confidence to speak up and speak out. There are times when clients, usually males, will share those *jokes* and laugh it off like what was said couldn't possibly be hurtful because after all it was a *joke*...and we're friends.

Prior to attending school for massage, I attended a predominantly white college. During my second year, while I was walking to work, a car full of white males drove slowly alongside me on the street. They shouted, "Go back to the zoo, you fucking monkey!" and threw a glass beer bottle at my head before speeding off. This was 2004, supposedly a time when racism no longer existed.

Why did I recall this memory? Because that, to me, is outward racism. So obvious that no one would question their intentions or classify it as a joke. So when a white person shared a *joke* about black people to me, a black person, that was supposed to be funny, my initial emotion wasn't rage like it was when a bottle was thrown at my head. Quite frankly, I was more overwhelmed with a feeling of disbelief that the person would feel comfortable enough to share such a story with racial undertones.

I learned many things about myself while working in the massage room. Apparently when in shock, I clam up instead of rage. Again, those clients are few and far between. In fact, it's more likely that someone will insert their foot into their mouth when they think they're in similar company. I've never heard a client make a outwardly racist statement about a black person, but I've heard enough comments about Mexicans, gays, and Middle Eastern people that, for a while, I believed that all white people held racist beliefs against every race imaginable. They just needed the privacy to admit it freely.

What bothered me more than the possibility of a client ever being stupid enough to do or say anything offensive in the room was the assumption that I've experienced it. It never failed. I never had a black person ask me if clients were racist, but every white receptionist at every place I worked always asked me this question. Lots of white massage therapists asked this question. Which led me to believe it was probably happening more often than I really knew. Maybe they were hearing things on the other side of the phone or in the privacy of their rooms that I was not privileged to hear.

One receptionist made it a point to inform me every time a client referred to me as *the black girl* because they couldn't remember my name. Well, my name is hard to pronounce to some and as long as the money made it to my pocket, I didn't care what description they gave as long as it was not offensive. The last time I checked, I am black, so to be described as such does not offend me.

✳

It was just one week after the election in 2008. I remember the day vividly because I had just said goodbye to one of my regular unicorns. She was a rarity in those parts. It wasn't very often that we had black clients in the spa, let alone a regular. But she was mine. I remember greeting her in the lobby and we had our normal small talk heading back to the room. As soon as I closed the door, she embraced me and said, "Can you believe it?"

I didn't even need to ask what she was talking about because I already knew. It didn't occur to me until many years later that we felt it necessary to celebrate in private. Our excitement over having our first black president wasn't something that we could enjoy openly. The owner of the spa was a strong

Republican. She'd spent the past few months openly sharing her distaste for President Obama during the campaign. Those of us who voted for him were definitely in the minority in this place. After the election, the owner strongly advised that no one discuss politics on the job. Go figure.

I smiled from ear to ear in the privacy of the massage room. We whispered excitedly but kept our voices down and spent the entire hour of her massage talking about the history that was being made. We shared our own stories, experiences, and hopes of changes to come. The massage ended, and I hugged her goodbye and quickly flipped my room.

At this spa, we were granted 15 minutes between sessions to allow us enough time to clean our room, grab something to eat, use the restroom, or just relax a little bit. It was also because we were the only spa in town that gave full 60-minute sessions. Other places give "spa hours" which is only 50 minutes on the table so all sessions could begin at the top of the hour.

During my 15-minute break that day, I was on cloud 9. I had never connected with a client on that level because most of them couldn't understand the black side of my world. So, understandably, I was happy.

※

It was time for my next appointment. I walked to the front to greet Mrs. White and introduced myself. She stared at me with a look that I couldn't comprehend in the moment. She rose slowly and seemed as though she wanted to finish her coffee. I offered to bring it back for her, but she refused.

"Is this your first time here?"

"Yes."

"I see from your paperwork it's also your first massage. I always tell people the first massage is like an introduction to an addiction you never knew you had." I laughed to lighten the mood. She seemed uptight, and usually a bit of humor helps. It did nothing to lighten Mrs. White's mood.

I'd given this speech countless times on the way back to the room. I always time it perfectly so that we were in the room by the time I finished the statement, "Go ahead and step in." Mrs. White stepped past me and sat in the client chair in the corner of the room, holding firmly onto her purse. "So are there any areas you would like me to focus on today?"

"Um, no, not really. My daughter got me a gift certificate last year, and I needed to use it before it expired."

"I understand. Well since there aren't any areas bothering you, I'll just do a full body today and spend a little extra time on your back. Most people like more time there. Since this is your first time getting a massage, I'll explain things a bit. I'll step out of the room to allow you to undress to your level of comfort. That just means if you want to leave your underwear on, you can," I said, placing my hand on my backside. "Once you're undressed, you'll just climb right in between this sheet and blanket." I lifted the top sheet and blanket slightly and swept my hand between the sheets. "Everything in the room is adjustable. The lights, music volume, and even the temperature on the table can be adjusted. If it's too warm, too bright, or too loud just let me know. Feel free to let me know about pressure as well. If it's too deep or not deep enough, don't hesitate to speak up." I gave a friendly smile. "Do you have any questions?"

"No," she mumbled.

"Okay! I'll step out so you can undress. Just climb right in between these sheets and lie face up for me. I'll give you a few minutes, and I'll knock before I come back in." I left the room and closed the door gently.

I headed back to the employee break room, washed my hands, and wrapped them in a warm towel. The first massage is often the most memorable. Even if you waited until you were in your late 60s, like Mrs. White. I always wanted the first touch to be warm. Cold hands are a shock to the system. When you're on a massage table and everything is warm, the last thing you need are cold hands abruptly jolting you from the relaxed state.

I tapped on the door three times and cracked it just a bit. "All set?"

"Yes." Her voice was muffled. When I arrived back in the room, she was lying face down underneath everything she could lift. Normally if the client misunderstands and lies face down instead of face up, I just let them stay there and adjust my massage so they don't feel any type of embarrassment. But this was far from right.

She was lying directly on the heating apparatus. She was under a blanket, two flat sheets, and three full-length body towels that were a barrier between the heating apparatus and the first flat sheet. I needed her to move.

"Oops. Looks like you went too far. I'm going to step out again for a second so you can adjust. You'll want to lie right here between these two sheets." I separated them again with my hands, so she could see what I meant.

"Oh, well you didn't say, so I didn't know what to do."

"No worries. I'll just step out so you're not directly on the warmer. I'll be right outside the door, so give a holler when you're ready for me to come back in." I stepped out and heard Mrs. White shuffling through the door. When the noise and movements stopped, I waited a few seconds before I tapped lightly on the door again. I opened it just a crack. "All set?"

"Yes," she grumbled.

"Okay. That's better. Are you warm enough?"

"You can turn that thing off."

"No problem." I pushed the button three times until it let out a long beep, indicating the table warmer was off. "How's the music and lighting for you?"

"It's fine." She was scowling, and I assumed it was

because she was completely out of her relaxed state from having to get up from the table and readjust.

I removed my dish of massage cream from the hot towel cabinet on the trolley next to the table. I placed my hands gently on her shoulders, slowly pressing them into the table with each exhale she made, to try and help her relax. My initial touch caused her to shudder. I assumed she was nervous since it was her first massage. After a few breaths and failed attempts to get her to relax by pressing on her shoulders, I cradled her head with one hand and placed the other on her forehead. Surely the warmth of my hands would calm her nervous spirit. No luck.

I began working on her neck, which she held so stiffly that I could barely turn her head to the side. Stiffness was common during first massages. Clients have a tendency to want to hold their head and limbs up for you, to "help." It's not necessary and is very counterproductive to what we are trying to do. But Mrs. White wasn't helping, she was resisting. With every touch, she retracted and pulled away, almost as if she didn't want me to touch her.

She laid on the table, with her eyes wide open and staring at the ceiling. "Are you comfortable?" I asked, just loud enough to be heard over the music playing in the speakers.

"It's fine." I didn't believe her. She looked uncomfortable, but at this point, there was nothing I could do. She wasn't giving me much to work with, nor was she willing to offer more than two-word answers. I finished working her neck and shoulders and headed to one of her arms.

"How's the pressure? I can adjust if you need." I was hoping for a sign that she was enjoying her session.

"It's fine." I figured.

The next ten minutes felt like 30. Not because she didn't speak but because she recoiled at every point of contact. She watched my hands touch her arms and when she noticed herself watching, forced herself to stare only at the ceiling. It wasn't until I made it to her legs that she began to relax. Had I known the way the rest of the massage would end, I would have preferred the silent recoils.

Before I worked on my clients' legs, I would wrap their feet in hot towels. It served two purposes. If there was any dirt, lint, or odor, hot towels took away some of the *ick*. They also added that little something extra. It was inexplicable, but I remember the first time someone used hot towels on my feet. At the time, I hadn't received a lot of massages yet, but I loved when hot towels were used on my feet. From that point on, I always used them in my sessions.

For Mrs. White, it seemed like those hot towels transformed her into a whole new person. I could feel her entire body relax and let go through her feet. And let go she did. In that hour, she let go of everything that she had been holding in for years.

"That feels heavenly."

I knew better than to speak. There was nothing,

really, for me to say. I knew it felt good. Instead, I smiled and hoped she could hear the good vibes and relief I felt because she was finally enjoying her first massage.

"I don't know why I waited so long to try this."

"It's better late than never."

"My daughter bought me this gift certificate last year for Christmas. I set it in a drawer and forgot all about it. You know, the drawer everyone has that just collects every little old thing. Last week, something told me to clean that old thing out and there it was. I saw the date and thought, *If I don't use this, she's gonna be so mad.*"

I laughed softly to acknowledge I was listening.

"In my day, people didn't do this…massage. You'd go and get your hair done and that was all. Now you all do your nails and *massage*. How long have you done this?"

"A few years." I was never comfortable telling anyone I had only been licensed for less than 2 years. A few years just sounded better.

"You're wonderful."

"Thank you."

"Do you have to go to school for this?"

"Yes. My program was 12 months. Most programs are between 9 and 18 months."

"Interesting. Do your hands ever get tired?"

"Sometimes. But after a while, you just get in shape for it." I smiled, having lost count of the number of times I had answered that question.

The silence continued for a few minutes, and Mrs. White seemed to go into a trance.

"Yes, things are definitely different nowadays. Can you imagine a black president?"

I wasn't sure where she was going with it, so I said, "Yeah, this is certainly historical."

"I voted for him, you know."

"Hmm," I mumbled to acknowledge I heard her.

"Things are different now. In my time, things were just different. Coloreds couldn't do anything. You'd never expect one to become president. Back then, things were just so different."

I continued the massage, in disbelief that she would so casually refer to us as *coloreds*, but I didn't interrupt.

"I remember they couldn't even eat with us or share a water fountain."

I wondered if the *they* she was speaking of had much darker skin than me. Maybe she had gone color-blind in her old age and didn't realize I was one of them. Still I said nothing.

"My friends and I would go to our favorite restaurant every day. Once, a colored boy was there. He came and just sat. Didn't say a word. We were so angry. My friends and I yelled and shouted the meanest things at him, but he still wouldn't leave. Oh, we threw food and drinks. Spat at him and called him all types of names. And he just sat there. Oh, that made my friend so angry. He shoved him onto the floor and we gave him a few good kicks. My friend lifted that colored boy up by his shirt and dragged him right outside the door. We threw more food and shouted until he ran on down the street. I never felt right about what we did. I knew it was wrong. But I was right there with them. Sometimes I wonder what happened to that colored boy. It was different then."

She paused longer, for what felt like an eternity. Somehow, my hands continued moving while I sat at her feet in silence. I had read stories, saw pictures, and heard my grandparents share their accounts about how things were *back then*. I never imagined I would be sitting at the feet of evil.

Had someone told me this was how the session was going to be, I could have sworn on my life that I would curse this woman out and end the session. You never think something like this will happen to you. When it does, words, emotions, and all logical thought processes seem to disappear. During the pause, she no longer existed. Only the thoughts and images of a man she'd assaulted.

While my hands were clearly on autopilot, my mind had drifted back in time to a black and white replay of her and three friends attacking an innocent man, all because those were the times. That's the excuse I had heard for many years when my white coworkers would share stories of clients making racist remarks in the room. I'd get angry with them, and they'd always say, "It's not their fault. They aren't really racist. They just grew up in a different time."

But here I was. Hands still selling out, defying my

emotions, ignoring my anger. My hands still moved. Then the long pause ended.

"I'm sorry."

Those two words never landed harder on my ears. Mrs. White had unloaded the burden she had been carrying within for the past 50 or so years. My hands still moved. I never acknowledged her apology. Instead, I lifted the blanket and asked her to turn over. It was time for the second half of her massage.

I had visions of the man Mrs. White and her friends assaulted. I wondered if he would accept her apology. I wondered where he was now. Was he an activist? Would another therapist have spoken up? Ended the session? Asked her to stop talking? Why were my hands betraying me and accepting the things I'd sworn I would never put up with in the treatment room? I felt empty inside. Emotionally drained.

After the massage, I left the treatment room without a word. I didn't ask how she was feeling. I didn't let her know the session was over. I didn't tell her know she could take as much time as she needed getting off the table to get dressed. I didn't say that I would meet her outside the room with a bottle of water. Though my hands moved, my mouth did not.

They say a strong woman uses her voice. If that is true, then I was weak. I went to the break room, washed my hands, and cried with no privacy. I couldn't find the words to explain why the exchange was so powerful. How do you explain to a room full of white coworkers that you didn't know what to say?

How do you explain the anger that you feel on behalf of another person who is not you? How do you explain to another black person why your body continued the session when your mind had nothing left to give? I didn't know how, so I didn't try. Instead, I sat crouched in a corner, feeling helpless and powerless.

The tears eventually dried, my coworkers stopped asking what was wrong, and my legs regained the strength to stand. I returned to my treatment room and removed the soiled sheets from the past hour.

I eventually found the words I could not speak, though I still don't have the answers for why. But I do truly believe that people are guided to the best table for them. And it doesn't always have to do with the massage.

Don't miss…..

Success Of A Failed Therapist

And next…

Shift

available September 2018.

TOUCHED

114